USING

VITAMIN C

FOR BEGINNERS

Unlocking Vital Health Benefits For Optimal Wellness, Skin Health, Boost Immunity And More

DR. SPARKS RUBIO

Copyright © Sparks Rubio, 2023

All rights reserved. No part of this book may be reproduced or transmitted in any form or by any means, electronic or mechanical, including photocopying, recording, or by any information storage and retrieval system, without permission in writing from the author, except for brief quotations embodied in critical reviews and certain other noncommercial uses permitted by copyright law.

DISCLAIMER

The information presented in this book is intended for general informational purposes only. It is not a substitute for professional medical advice, diagnosis, or treatment.

The author and publisher of this book have made every effort to ensure that the information provided is accurate and up-to-date at the time of publication. However, medical and scientific knowledge is constantly evolving, and new research may emerge. Therefore, the information in this book should not be considered a definitive source for medical or nutritional advice.

It is essential to consult with a qualified healthcare professional before making any decisions.

The author and publisher disclaim any liability for any adverse outcomes or consequences resulting from the use or misuse of the information in this book. Readers are urged to use their discretion and judgment when making decisions about their health and wellness.

By reading this book, you agree to do so at your own risk and should not use it as a substitute for professional medical advice or treatment.

TABLE OF CONTENTS

INTRODUCTION TO VITAMIN C.................................9

THE IMPORTANCE OF VITAMIN C 9

THE AIM AND EXTENT OF THIS BOOK 11

HOW TO UTILIZE THIS MANUAL........................14

CHAPTER ONE 18

VITAMIN C DEFINITIOM 18

FUNDAMENTALS OF VITAMINS 18

KNOWING ABOUT VITAMIN C............................19

HISTORICAL CONTEXT 22

CHAPTER TWO 26

ADVANTAGES OF VITAMIN C FOR HEALTH 26

IMMUNE SYSTEM SUPPORT..................................27

SKIN HEALTH AND BEAUTY 28

COGNITIVE FUNCTION 31

FURTHER POSSIBLE ADVANTAGES 32

CHAPTER THREE 34

VITAMIN C SOURCES VIA DIET 34

ORGANIC FOOD SUPPLIES..................................34

DIETARY ALLOWANCE THAT IS............................36

FACTORS INFLUENCING FOODS' VITAMIN C........39

CHAPTER FOUR 44

INSUFFICIENCY OF VITAMIN C 44

SYMPTOMS AND INDICATIONS.............................44

GROUPS AT RISK 48

CONDITIONS ASSOCIATED WITH DEFICIENCY.......50

CHAPTER FIVE 52

TYPES OF SUPPLEMENTAL VITAMIN C 52

SODIUM ASCORBATE 53

ESTER-C 55

LIPOSOMAL VITAMIN C..56

CHOOSING THE CORRECT FORM 57

CHAPTER SIX 60

TAKING VITAMIN C SUPPLEMENTS............................60

SUGGESTED DOSES 60

SAFETY AND TOLERABILITY 62

DRUG INTERACTIONS..64

PARTICULAR TAKEAWAYS (CHILDREN, THE
ELDERLY, AND PREGNANCY) 65

CHAPTER SEVEN..68

IMMUNITY AND VITAMIN C..68

HOW IMMUNE FUNCTION IS SUPPORTED.............69

THE ROLE OF VITAMIN C IN PREVENTING............70

OTHER IMMUNE BENEFITS 71

CHAPTER EIGHT 74

VITAMIN C AND SKIN CARE................................74

COLLAGEN PRODUCTION................................74

SKIN AGING AND WRINKLES 75

TOPICAL VITAMIN C PRODUCTS.....................76

CHAPTER NINE 80

VITAMIN C AND CHRONIC DISEASES......................80

CARDIOVASCULAR DISEASES 81

CANCER 82

OSTEOARTHRITIS 84

AGE-RELATED MACULAR DEGENERATION............85

CHAPTER TEN...88

VITAMIN C AND MENTAL HEALTH 88

ROLE IN BRAIN HEALTH...............................88

DEPRESSION AND ANXIETY 90

COGNITIVE DECLINE.....................................92

CHAPTER ELEVEN 96

VITAMIN C AND ATHLETES...................................96

EXERCISE AND OXIDATIVE STRESS 96

BENEFITS FOR ATHLETES.................................98

DOSAGE AND TIMING 100

CHAPTER TWELVE 104

RISKS AND SIDE EFFECTS..........................104

SIDE EFFECTS OF HIGH DOSES 104

ALLERGIES AND SENSITIVITIES 108

POSSIBLE DANGERS 112

CHAPTER THIRTEEN 116

VITAMIN C AND OTHER NUTRIENTS 116

VITAMIN C AND IRON ABSORPTION 117

VITAMIN C AND VITAMIN D.............................119

SYNERGISTIC NUTRIENT COMBINATIONS...........120

CHAPTER FOURTEEN..................................124

HOW TO PICK A REPUTABLE SOURCE OF VITAMIN C
....124

CONCLUSION 129

YUMMY RECIPES TO INCREASE YOUR CONSUMPTION
OF VITAMIN C 129

VITAMIN C'S FUNCTION IN YOUR HEALTH..........131

INTRODUCTION TO VITAMIN C

THE IMPORTANCE OF VITAMIN C

Amidst the plethora of nutrients, minerals, and vitamins found on the planet, Vitamin C stands out as exceptional and important, well acknowledged for its vital role in preserving human health. This water-soluble vitamin, sometimes referred to as ascorbic acid, is well-known for its antioxidant qualities as well as its critical role in numerous physiological processes. It is essential for the production of collagen, a structural protein that is necessary for the development of bones, connective tissues, blood vessels, and skin.

Moreover, vitamin C can effectively scavenge free radicals, thereby shielding our DNA and cells from oxidative damage.

Vitamin C is well-known for its ability to strengthen the immune system in addition to its functions as an antioxidant and collagen-forming substance. By encouraging the synthesis of white blood cells, which are essential for fending off infections and illnesses, it fortifies the immune system. Furthermore, vitamin C is essential for vegetarians and vegans because it helps the body absorb non-heme iron, which is the kind of iron present in plant-based diets.

Vitamin C is important for reasons other than these health advantages. Its potential to lower the risk of chronic illnesses like cardiovascular disease and to improve general well-being have both been studied. Vitamin C has a vital role in human health, as seen by its involvement in preventing scurvy, a condition historically linked to a deficit in the vitamin.

THE AIM AND EXTENT OF THIS BOOK

Our goal in writing this book is to provide readers with a thorough grasp of vitamin C's function in health and wellness. We have carefully selected a plethora of information to serve as a comprehensive guide to understanding, applying, and reaping the benefits of vitamin C. This book appeals to a wide range of readers, including health enthusiasts, medical professionals, and those looking for helpful suggestions on incorporating Vitamin C into their daily lives.

This book has three goals in mind. First and foremost, it seeks to inform readers of the critical role that vitamin C plays in the body, elucidating its complex processes and its wider implications for maintaining health. Second, to help people make educated food choices and guarantee an appropriate intake of this crucial nutrient, it aims to offer useful insights into the dietary sources of Vitamin C. Lastly, this book explores vitamin C's possible therapeutic uses, including how it can be used to prevent and treat a range of illnesses.

This book covers a wide range of subjects, such as the discovery of vitamin C's history, its biochemical characteristics, suggested dietary allowances, and its application in the prevention and treatment of medical disorders. To assist readers in making well-informed decisions about how to include this nutrient in their everyday lives, we will examine the sources of vitamin C, both natural and supplemental. We'll also go over the most recent study on vitamin C's possible medicinal uses, including immune support, skin care, and other areas.

HOW TO UTILIZE THIS MANUAL

To get the most out of this extensive book, you must know how to browse it and make appropriate use of the information it contains. This book's structure makes it easy for readers to follow along, with each section building on the one before it to provide a coherent and seamless flow of information. It is recommended that readers approach this guide with an open mind and a curiosity to learn about the world of vitamin C, from its historical background to its contemporary uses.

Although there are no hard and fast guidelines for using this book, we advise beginning with the chapters that most closely correspond with your present requirements or interests. For example, the first several chapters will be especially informative if you're looking for broad information regarding the significance of vitamin C. You are welcome to skip to the sections on skincare and immune support, for example, if those are the applications that most interest you. This book is meant to be a versatile and adaptive tool for your path to improved health and well-being.

To sum up, the pages that follow will be devoted to revealing the complex tale of vitamin C. We hope that as you go on this exploration of ascorbic acid, the knowledge you gain will be useful and illuminating, enabling you to make decisions about your health and well-being that are well-informed.

CHAPTER ONE

VITAMIN C DEFINITIOM

FUNDAMENTALS OF VITAMINS

Vitamins are vital organic substances that our systems need in trace amounts to sustain different physiological processes and general well-being. These molecules serve as coenzymes, or substances that help enzymes catalyze chemical reactions in the body, and as such, they are vital to metabolic processes. The two primary categories of vitamins are fat-soluble and water-soluble. Water-soluble vitamins, such as vitamin C, dissolve in water and are not significantly retained by the body. Conversely, fat-soluble vitamins have a longer shelf life and are kept in fatty tissues.

KNOWING ABOUT VITAMIN C

Ascorbic acid, another name for vitamin C, is a water-soluble vitamin that is essential to several bodily metabolic processes. Since our bodies are unable to produce it, we must get it from our diets as it is thought to be vital for human health. Well known for its antioxidant qualities, vitamin C helps shield cells from oxidative stress and cellular damage brought on by free radicals, which are unstable molecules.

The manufacture of collagen, a structural protein essential to the health of our skin, cartilage, tendons, and blood vessels, is one of the most well-known uses of vitamin C. Scurvy, which is characterized by weak blood vessels, bleeding gums, and joint discomfort, is one of the disorders caused by the body's inability to manufacture collagen without vitamin C. Due to a shortage of fresh produce on lengthy sea trips, scurvy was once a common ailment among sailors.

In the digestive tract, vitamin C is also necessary for the absorption of non-heme iron, or iron derived from plant sources. It changes iron into a form that is easier for the body to absorb, which is essential in avoiding iron deficiency anemia. This is especially crucial for people who eat a vegetarian or vegan diet because the body absorbs iron from plant sources less easily.

Additionally, vitamin C is essential for the immunological system. It has been linked to improving white blood cell function, which is in charge of defending the body against illnesses. Supplementing with vitamin C may help lessen the duration and intensity of the common cold, according to certain research.

Vitamin C is also well known for its capacity to lower blood pressure and improve blood vessel function, therefore lowering the risk of heart disease and other chronic illnesses. Research in this area is ongoing, but it might also play a part in lowering the risk of some cancers.

HISTORICAL CONTEXT

The history of vitamin C is intimately linked to the study of scurvy, the condition brought on by a lack of it. A major worry for sailors in the 15th and 16th centuries during the Age of Exploration was scurvy. Extended maritime expeditions frequently led to a scarcity of fresh produce, resulting in scurvy epidemics among seamen. Symptoms of this illness included weakness, exhaustion, bleeding swollen gums, and in extreme cases, even death.

One of the first controlled studies to look into the relationship between scurvy and other dietary components was carried out in the eighteenth century by the Scottish navy surgeon James Lind. He discovered that scurvy could be effectively prevented and treated with citrus fruits like lemons and limes. With this discovery, our knowledge of vitamin C's therapeutic benefits began to take shape.

Ascorbic acid, an isolated chemical substance, was discovered to be the active component in citrus fruits that prevents scurvy only in the 20th century. Albert Szent-Gyorgyi, a Hungarian scientist, was granted the Nobel Prize in Physiology or Medicine in 1932 in recognition of his research on vitamin C. Since then, the significance of vitamin C for human nutrition and health has gained widespread recognition.

Vitamin C is an essential ingredient that is needed for several physiological processes, such as the synthesis of collagen, the maintenance of the immune system, and the avoidance of scurvy.

Its discovery that it can prevent and treat scurvy has altered our understanding of this vital vitamin and is associated with historical significance.

CHAPTER TWO

ADVANTAGES OF VITAMIN C FOR HEALTH

Ascorbic acid, another name for vitamin C, is a water soluble vitamin that is essential for many aspects of health and well-being. This important vitamin is well-known for its many advantages, which include immune system support, antioxidant qualities, and even contributions to skin, wound healing, cardiovascular, eye, and cognitive health, among other possible benefits.

Vitamin C has strong antioxidant properties, which means it helps shield the body from the harm that free radicals can cause. Highly reactive chemicals known as free radicals can harm DNA, proteins, and cells, which accelerates aging and several chronic diseases. Vitamin C functions as an antioxidant, scavenging free radicals to counteract their damaging effects and lessen oxidative stress in the body. This characteristic is essential for preserving general health and lowering the risk of chronic illnesses.

IMMUNE SYSTEM SUPPORT

It is commonly known that vitamin C helps to support the immune system. It improves the generation and functionality of immune cells, including lymphocytes and white blood cells. Additionally, it can improve how well the body's defense systems react to infections and illnesses. Frequent vitamin C intake may lessen the intensity and length of respiratory infections, such as the common cold.

SKIN HEALTH AND BEAUTY

Vitamin C is necessary for the synthesis of collagen, a protein that gives the skin, hair, and nails structure. Getting enough vitamin C encourages the production of collagen, which keeps the skin supple and keeps wrinkles from appearing.

It also helps with scar healing and skin restoration. Because of its capacity to lessen hyper pigmentation and enhance skin texture, vitamin C is a common ingredient in skincare products.

Vitamin C is essential for both tissue repair and wound healing. It promotes the growth of collagen and the creation of new blood vessels, both of which are necessary for healthy wound healing. In wounds that have enough vitamin C, healing occurs more quickly and leaves fewer scars. This characteristic is especially crucial for wound healing and surgical recuperation.

Research has indicated that vitamin C may have a role in maintaining cardiovascular health. By increasing blood vessel flexibility and lowering the risk of atherosclerosis a disorder marked by the accumulation of plaque in arteries it aids in the maintenance of healthy blood vessels. In addition, vitamin C functions as an anti-inflammatory and blood pressure-lowering agent, lowering the risk of heart disease.

Vitamin C is also involved in maintaining eye health. One of the main causes of vision loss in older persons is age-related macular degeneration (AMD), which it can help avoid. The antioxidant characteristics of vitamin C can help reduce the oxidative stress and inflammation linked to AMD. Additionally, vitamin C helps to maintain the health of the blood vessels in the eyes, which improves eyesight.

COGNITIVE FUNCTION

New research indicates that vitamin C might be important for preserving cognitive function, especially in older people. It is believed that diseases like Alzheimer's disease and cognitive decline are related to oxidative stress and inflammation. Antioxidant qualities of vitamin C may shield the brain from these damaging processes, thereby delaying cognitive aging.

FURTHER POSSIBLE ADVANTAGES

In addition to the previously listed, well-researched advantages, vitamin C may also help prevent cancer, lower the incidence of gout, and enhance iron absorption a crucial process for those who suffer from iron deficiency anemia. It might also help the body's reaction to allergies and asthma, as well as maintaining lung health.

Vitamin C is a flexible nutrient that offers several health advantages. It is a vital part of a balanced diet because of its anti-oxidant qualities, immune system support, effects on skin and wound healing, cardiovascular and eye health, and other possible benefits. Keeping general health and well-being can be achieved by taking supplements or eating foods high in vitamin C.

CHAPTER THREE

VITAMIN C SOURCES VIA DIET

ORGANIC FOOD SUPPLIES

Ascorbic acid, another name for vitamin C, is a substance that is vital to human health. It is essential for wound healing, immune system function, and iron absorption from plant-based diets. It's critical to get enough sources of vitamin C in your diet to stay healthy. Thankfully, a wide range of natural food sources include vitamin C.

One of the most well-known forms of vitamin C is found in citrus fruits. Nutrient-dense fruits and vegetables include oranges, grapefruits, lemons, and limes. All the vitamin C you need each day can be found in only one medium-sized orange. In addition, additional fruits high in vitamin C include papaya, guava, strawberries, and kiwi.

Besides fruits, veggies also provide a significant amount of vitamin C. Bell peppers are well-known for having a high vitamin C content, especially the red and green types. More vitamin C can be found in one cup of raw red bell pepper than in an orange. Significant levels of vitamin C are also present in other vegetables, including spinach, kale, broccoli, and Brussels sprouts.

In addition to being delicious, berries like raspberries, blueberries, and strawberries are great providers of this important vitamin. They can be eaten on their own, as a topping for cereal and desserts, or blended into smoothies.

DIETARY ALLOWANCE THAT IS RECOMMENDED

The recommended daily intake of vitamin C for humans to maintain optimal health is known as the Recommended Dietary Allowance (RDA). The RDA is typically determined to meet the needs of the majority of the population, while it varies based on factors such as age, sex, and life stage. The RDA for vitamin C, as of the cutoff date in 2021, is as follows:

1. Babies:

- For 0–6 months: 40 mg daily

- For 7 to 12 months: 50 mg daily

2. Little ones:

- Ages 1-3: 15 mg daily

- 4–8 years old: 25 mg daily

- Ages 9 to 13: 45 mg daily

3. Teenagers and Adults:

- For males aged 14 to 18, 75 mg daily

- For girls aged 14 to 18, 65 mg daily

• Males aged 19 and up 90 mg daily

• 75 mg daily for females 19 years of age and above

4. Women who are expecting or nursing:

• Teens (14–18 years old) who are pregnant: 80 mg daily

• Adults (19 years of age and older) who are pregnant: 85 mg daily

• Teens (14–18 years old) who are nursing: 115 mg daily

• Adults 19 years of age and above who are lactating: 120 mg daily

These recommended daily allowances (RDAs) are made to prevent vitamin

C deficiency, which can cause scurvy, a disease marked by weakening in the muscles, swollen and bleeding gums, and weariness. The actual amount required, however, can vary depending on several factors, such as lifestyle choices, illnesses, and individual metabolism.

FACTORS INFLUENCING FOODS' VITAMIN C CONTENT

To make sure you're getting the most out of your dietary sources of vitamin C, it's important to understand the various factors that can affect the amount of vitamin C in foods. The following are some of the major variables influencing food's vitamin C content:

1. Storage and Handling: Oxygen, heat, and light can all affect vitamin C. Vitamin C concentration in fruits and vegetables can be preserved by storing them in cool, dark settings with minimal exposure to air. Moreover, boiling and other similar cooking techniques might cause some vitamin C to be lost because it can seep into the cooking liquid.

2. Ripeness: As fruits and vegetables ripen, their vitamin C content might vary. It's a good idea to eat fruits and vegetables as fresh as possible

because they might often lose vitamin C when they ripen.

3. Processing: The amount of vitamin C in food can be affected by how it is prepared. Vitamin C degrading effects can result from canning, freezing, and drying. Foods that are fresh and lightly processed typically contain more vitamins C.

4. Seasonal Variations: Depending on the season, foods may contain different amounts of vitamin C. Vitamin C levels are generally higher in fruits and vegetables that are harvested during their peak season than in those that are harvested out of season or stored for long periods.

5. Cooking Techniques: The amount of vitamin C in food might vary depending on the cooking technique used. Generally speaking, steaming or microwaving veggies preserves more vitamin C than boiling them. Achieving a balance between retaining the vitamin C content and boiling out possible germs is crucial.

6. Soil Quality: Crops' vitamin C concentration is influenced by the nutrients in the soil. More nutrient-dense fruits and vegetables can result from soil that is high in important minerals and nutrients.

Vitamin C comes from a range of natural food sources and is a necessary ingredient for supporting general health. The Recommended Dietary Allowance (RDA) for vitamin C varies depending on age and stage of life, so make sure your diet has enough of the vitamin to avoid insufficiency. You may also make the most of your dietary choices and maintain a sufficient intake of vitamin C for optimal health by being aware of the factors such as storage, ripeness, processing, seasonal fluctuations, cooking methods, and soil quality that affect the vitamin C concentration in foods.

CHAPTER FOUR

INSUFFICIENCY OF VITAMIN C

Ascorbic acid, another name for vitamin C, is a water-soluble vitamin that is essential to many body processes. Scurvy, or a vitamin C deficiency, can cause a variety of symptoms and health problems. We will go into great detail about vitamin C deficiency symptoms and signs, at-risk categories, and illnesses related to this deficiency in this talk.

SYMPTOMS AND INDICATIONS

The production of collagen, a structural protein critical to the integrity of connective tissues, skin, and blood vessels, depends on vitamin C. Therefore, collagen dysfunction is linked to the main symptoms and indicators of vitamin C deficiency. These may consist of:

1. Fatigue and Weakness: People who are deficient in vitamin C may have ongoing fatigue and weakness, which can make it difficult for them to go about their everyday lives. This is frequently among the first indications of scurvy.

2. Gum Issues: Classic indications of scurvy include bleeding and swollen gums. This happens because the health of the gums' connective tissues

and blood vessels depends on vitamin C.

3. Skin Problems: The skin could get rough, dry, and prone to bruising easily. There may also be signs of slow wound healing and the growth of tiny red or purple patches called petechiae.

4. Joint Pain: Weakened connective tissues resulting from a vitamin C deficit can cause joint pain and stiffness. It's possible to have stiff, achy joints.

5. Anemia: Anemia can occur in cases of severe vitamin C deficiency. This happens because iron absorption is hampered without vitamin C, which

helps with the absorption of non-heme iron from plant-based diets.

6. Swollen and Painful Joints: Vitamin C insufficiency may occasionally result in swollen and painful joints. Children are especially prone to this.

7. Muscle Weakness: Insufficient vitamin C can cause muscles' structural integrity to be damaged, leading to the development of muscular weakness.

8. Weight Loss: People who experience unexplained weight loss may be deficient in vitamin C, as they may experience appetite loss and digestive difficulties.

Because vitamin-rich foods are readily available, vitamin C insufficiency is comparatively uncommon in modern nations; yet, several groups continue to be at increased risk:

1. Bad Diet: People who don't eat enough of the main sources of vitamin C, fruits, and vegetables, run the risk of being deficient. This is particularly valid for people who don't have easy access to fresh fruit.

2. Smokers: The body needs more vitamin C when smoking, thus to maintain healthy levels, smokers may require higher doses of the vitamin.

3. Chronic Illness: Individuals who suffer from long-term conditions including cancer, gastrointestinal issues, or renal disease may require more vitamin C or have less absorption, which puts them at risk.

4. Alcoholism: Drinking too much alcohol might impede the body's ability to absorb and use vitamin C, raising the possibility of a deficit.

5. Infants: Infants who are breastfed by moms who are deficient in vitamin C or who are fed formula lacking in vitamin C may be in danger.

CONDITIONS ASSOCIATED WITH DEFICIENCY

Scurvy is a serious ailment that can develop from a vitamin C deficiency if treatment is not received. Scurvy is typified by the following conditions:

1. Anemia: Scurvy patients may experience anemia as a result of reduced iron absorption, which can cause weakness and exhaustion.

2. Skin Lesions: Ecchymoses (bruises), little red or purple spots on the skin called "petechiae," and dry, scaly skin are common side effects of scurvy.

3. Gums that bleed easily and become inflamed can result in painful, swollen gums.

4. Joint and Bone Problems: Fractures and osteoporosis are examples of abnormalities in the bone that can be brought on by weakening connective tissues.

5. Muscle Weakness: Degradation of connective tissue can lead to discomfort and muscular weakness.

Scurvy is the most severe sign of a vitamin C shortage, which can cause a variety of other symptoms and health problems.

CHAPTER FIVE

TYPES OF SUPPLEMENTAL VITAMIN C

Ascorbic acid, another name for vitamin C, is a necessary nutrient that is vital to many body processes. It is well known for strengthening the immune system and having antioxidant qualities. Although you can get enough vitamin C from your food, taking supplements is a handy method to be sure you get enough each day. But there are different kinds of vitamin C supplements out today, and each has certain qualities and advantages of its own.

The most popular and extensively utilized type of vitamin C supplement is ascorbic acid. This substance dissolves in water and is present in a wide variety of fruits and vegetables. This vitamin C form is very efficient and has a good bioavailability, which means the body can absorb it easily. Because ascorbic acid supplements come in a variety of forms, such as pills, capsules, and powders, people can easily select the one that best suits their needs.

SODIUM ASCORBATE

Sodium ascorbate is a less acidic type of vitamin C than ascorbic acid because it has been buffered. For those who have sensitive stomachs or feel uncomfortable when taking ascorbic acid, this makes it a better option. Additionally, sodium ascorbate has a high bioavailability and is soluble in water. The majority of individuals can tolerate it well, and it is frequently sold as powder or capsules.

Another buffered form of vitamin C is calcium ascorbate, which uses calcium as the buffer. This makes it a good choice for anyone who wants to take a calcium and vitamin C supplement. Compared to ascorbic acid, it is less harsh on the stomach, and calcium is a necessary mineral for strong bones. There are several supplement forms of this type of vitamin C, including powders and pills.

ESTER-C

Ester-C is a proprietary vitamin C supplement that includes metabolites and calcium ascorbate. It is praised for its capacity to give the body more sustained vitamin C action. Ester-C is a fantastic option for people with delicate digestive systems because of its reputation for having a mild effect on the stomach. It is promoted as a more gastrointestinal-friendly type of vitamin C and is frequently offered as a pill or capsule.

LIPOSOMAL VITAMIN C

Supplementing with liposomal vitamin C is a relatively recent concept. Vitamin C is encapsulated in microscopic lipid (fat) bubbles known as liposomes. This technique is thought to improve vitamin C absorption because the liposomes facilitate more effective vitamin transport to cells and shield the vitamin from deterioration in the digestive system. Liposomal vitamin C is therefore assumed to offer improved bioavailability, enabling smaller dosages to produce comparable results.

CHOOSING THE CORRECT FORM

Depending on personal tastes and requirements, the best form of vitamin C should be chosen. For most people, ascorbic acid is a dependable and affordable solution. Take into consideration sodium ascorbate, calcium ascorbate, or Ester-C if you have a sensitive stomach. One option for those looking for increased bioavailability is liposomal vitamin C. Furthermore, since certain vitamin C supplements contain additives or sources of possible allergens, it's critical to take into account any dietary restrictions or allergies.

Before beginning any new supplement regimen, it is best to speak with a healthcare provider. They can offer tailored advice based on your unique needs and health state. They can also offer advice on the right dosage to help you reach your desired health objectives. The vitamin C supplement you choose should ultimately be in line with your particular demands and preferences for health.

CHAPTER SIX

TAKING VITAMIN C SUPPLEMENTS

SUGGESTED DOSES

Ascorbic acid, another name for vitamin C, is a necessary nutrient that is critical for many body processes, such as collagen synthesis, immunological support, and antioxidant defense. The appropriate daily dose of vitamin C depends on factors such as age, gender, and individual medical requirements. The recommended dietary amount (RDA) for most healthy persons is around 90 mg for men and 75 mg for women. However, greater doses could be required in specific situations, such as illness or pregnancy.

To achieve their daily needs, people may occasionally decide to take vitamin C supplements. When using supplements, typical daily amounts fall between 500 and 2000 mg. Healthcare providers can decide on the appropriate dosage based on each patient's unique needs. It is significant to remember that taking too much vitamin C might have negative effects, such as diarrhea and other digestive problems. As such, it is crucial to take into account individual circumstances while figuring out the right dosage.

When taken by recommended dosages, vitamin C is usually regarded as safe. Vitamin C is effectively absorbed and utilized by the human body from both food sources and supplementation. On the other hand, overindulgence may result in negative side effects, chiefly gastrointestinal distress such as cramps and diarrhea. Reducing the dosage can usually alleviate these side effects, which are usually transient. The majority of people tolerate vitamin C supplements well, however before taking large amounts, people with a history of kidney stones or certain medical disorders should speak with a healthcare professional.

Since vitamin C is a water-soluble vitamin, too much of it is eliminated through the urine, lowering the possibility of toxicity. To prevent reaching dangerous levels, it is crucial to watch intake, particularly if using supplements. It's vital to let healthcare professionals know about vitamin C supplementation when having diagnostic procedures because it may affect the precision of several medical tests, like blood glucose measures.

Vitamin C has the potential to interact with several different drugs. For instance, it might prevent some medications like some antibiotics and blood thinners from being absorbed or working as intended. To be sure there are no possible interactions that can reduce the effectiveness of their prescription drugs, people taking them should talk to their doctors about vitamin C supplements. When a patient takes vitamin C supplements, medical providers may occasionally need to change the dosage of their prescriptions.

PARTICULAR TAKEAWAYS (CHILDREN, THE ELDERLY, AND PREGNANCY)

1. Pregnancy: To maintain both their health and the development of the fetus, pregnant women require more vitamin C. Generally speaking, pregnant women should consume more per day than non-pregnant adults do. While most expectant mothers can get enough vitamin C from a balanced diet, those who struggle to get enough may find that taking vitamin C supplements, when advised by a healthcare professional, is beneficial.

2. Kids: Although children's growth and development depend on vitamin

C, it's normally best to meet their daily needs with a well-balanced diet. For children in good health who have access to a range of fruits and vegetables, supplements are usually not required. However, pediatricians may suggest vitamin C pills in the right dosages in some situations, such as youngsters who have dietary limitations or fussy eaters.

3. Elderly: Dietary habits and nutritional absorption can alter as people age. Supplementation should be taken into consideration since certain older persons may be susceptible to vitamin C insufficiency. To find out if vitamin C supplements are required, elderly people should

talk to a healthcare professional about their dietary and nutritional needs.

Vitamin C is a necessary nutrient with a host of health advantages, and in some cases, taking supplements can be beneficial. But it's important to pay attention to prescribed dosages, be mindful of possible drug interactions, and take the special needs of special populations like the elderly, children, and pregnant women into account.

CHAPTER SEVEN

IMMUNITY AND VITAMIN C

One important nutrient that is well-known for helping immune function is vitamin C. Also referred to as ascorbic acid, this water-soluble vitamin has a variety of functions that support general health and strengthen the body's defenses against different infections. There are three main ways that Vitamin C affects immune function: the way it helps the immune system, how it helps treat and prevent colds, and other immune-boosting effects.

HOW IMMUNE FUNCTION IS SUPPORTED BY VITAMIN C

Vitamin C functions as an antioxidant to support immune function. Free radicals are dangerous substances that the immune system frequently comes into contact with and can harm or impair immune cells. Because of its antioxidant qualities, vitamin C helps the body fight off these free radicals and lessen oxidative stress. Consequently, immune cells can maintain their integrity and functionality, which strengthens their ability to fight off infections.

Moreover, Vitamin C is involved in the production and function of white blood cells, which are integral components of the immune system. It improves the body's defenses against infections by inducing the production of phagocytes, lymphocytes, and neutrophils. Vitamin C also aids in the synthesis of collagen, a structural protein that helps maintain the integrity of the skin and mucous membranes, serving as a physical barrier against pathogens.

THE ROLE OF VITAMIN C IN PREVENTING AND TREATING COLDS

The relationship between Vitamin C and the prevention and treatment of colds has been a subject of interest for several years. While it may not completely prevent the common cold, Vitamin C has been shown to reduce the duration and severity of cold symptoms. It does so by boosting the body's production of interferons and antibodies, essential elements of the immune response to viral infections. Additionally, Vitamin C's ability to support the function of the respiratory tract's mucous membranes can help prevent viruses from entering the body.

OTHER IMMUNE BENEFITS

Vitamin C has various other immune benefits beyond cold prevention. It aids in the formation of antibodies, which are vital components of the adaptive immune system that specifically target and neutralize pathogens. Furthermore, this vitamin helps the body absorb iron from plant-based sources, such as spinach and beans. Iron is essential for the production of hemoglobin, which carries oxygen to immune cells and tissues. Improved iron absorption can contribute to enhanced immune function.

In times of increased physical or psychological stress, such as during illness or exposure to environmental toxins, the body's demand for Vitamin C may also rise. Supplementing with Vitamin C in such situations can help support the immune system's ability to handle stress and fight off infections more effectively.

Vitamin C is a cornerstone of immune support due to its antioxidant properties, its role in enhancing white blood cell production, and its influence on the prevention and treatment of colds. Beyond these primary functions, it aids in antibody formation, improves iron absorption, and provides a buffer against stress-related immune challenges.

CHAPTER EIGHT

VITAMIN C AND SKIN CARE

COLLAGEN PRODUCTION

One of the key roles of Vitamin C in skin care is its impact on collagen production. Collagen is a crucial protein responsible for maintaining the skin's structure, elasticity, and overall youthful appearance. As we age, collagen production naturally decreases, leading to the formation of wrinkles, fine lines, and sagging skin. Vitamin C plays a pivotal role in the synthesis of collagen. It stimulates the fibroblast cells in the skin, which are responsible for producing collagen. This increased collagen production helps in maintaining skin firmness and suppleness. Regular application of Vitamin C to the skin can contribute to improved collagen levels, thus reducing the visible signs of aging.

SKIN AGING AND WRINKLES

Vitamin C is a potent antioxidant, and its ability to counteract the effects of oxidative stress is particularly valuable in the context of skin aging. Over time, the skin is exposed to various environmental stressors, such as UV radiation and pollution, which can lead to the formation of free radicals.

These free radicals cause cellular damage, leading to premature aging and the formation of wrinkles. Vitamin C's antioxidant properties help neutralize these free radicals, protecting the skin from their harmful effects. Additionally, Vitamin C can reduce the appearance of existing wrinkles by stimulating collagen production, as mentioned earlier, and by promoting skin cell turnover. As a result, it is an essential component of anti-aging skincare routines.

TOPICAL VITAMIN C PRODUCTS

Incorporating Vitamin C into your skincare routine is made easy through the availability of topical products.

These products come in various forms, such as serums, creams, and lotions, making it convenient for individuals to introduce this beneficial nutrient into their daily regimen. Topical Vitamin C products are formulated with different concentrations of the vitamin, allowing users to choose the right product for their skin type and concerns. However, it's important to note that not all Vitamin C products are created equal. The stability and effectiveness of Vitamin C in these products can vary. Look for formulations with L-ascorbic acid, which is the most biologically active form of Vitamin C.

When using topical Vitamin C products, it's recommended to apply them in the morning as part of your morning skincare routine. Vitamin C can provide an extra layer of protection against UV radiation and environmental stressors. Be sure to use sunscreen as well to complement the effects of Vitamin C and to prevent potential photosensitivity. The regular use of Vitamin C products can lead to a more radiant, even-toned complexion diminished fine lines, and a healthier skin barrier.

Vitamin C is a vital component of an effective skincare regimen, particularly when it comes to collagen production, combating skin aging, and reducing wrinkles. Topical Vitamin C products are readily available and can be customized to suit individual skincare needs. By integrating Vitamin C into your daily routine, you can enjoy the benefits of improved skin health and a more youthful appearance.

CHAPTER NINE

VITAMIN C AND CHRONIC DISEASES

Vitamin C, also known as ascorbic acid, is a vital water-soluble vitamin that plays a significant role in various physiological processes in the human body. Its antioxidant properties have led to extensive research on its potential role in preventing and mitigating chronic diseases, including cardiovascular diseases, cancer, osteoarthritis, and age-related macular degeneration.

CARDIOVASCULAR DISEASES

Cardiovascular diseases, such as heart disease and stroke, are among the leading causes of death worldwide. Vitamin C has been investigated for its potential protective role in reducing the risk of these conditions. One way in which vitamin C contributes to heart health is through its antioxidant properties. It helps neutralize free radicals that can damage blood vessels, which is an important factor in the development of atherosclerosis, a condition characterized by the buildup of plaque in the arteries. Moreover, vitamin C supports the synthesis of collagen, a protein that helps maintain the integrity of blood vessel walls. This may aid in preventing the development of aneurysms and maintaining healthy blood pressure. Although research on vitamin C and cardiovascular diseases has yielded mixed results, there is evidence to suggest that adequate vitamin C intake, primarily from fruits and vegetables, can contribute to a reduced risk of heart disease.

CANCER

Cancer is a complex group of diseases characterized by the uncontrolled growth of abnormal cells. The potential of vitamin C in cancer prevention and treatment has garnered considerable interest. As an antioxidant, vitamin C can help protect cells from oxidative damage that may lead to cancer. Additionally, it plays a role in the formation of collagen, which is essential for wound healing and tissue repair, making it relevant in the context of cancer treatment. Some studies have explored the use of high-dose intravenous vitamin C as an adjuvant therapy in cancer treatment, aiming to enhance the effectiveness of chemotherapy or radiation therapy. However, the evidence on the efficacy of vitamin C in cancer prevention and treatment is still inconclusive, and more research is needed to establish its role definitively.

OSTEOARTHRITIS

Osteoarthritis is a degenerative joint disease that causes pain, stiffness, and reduced joint mobility. Although osteoarthritis is primarily associated with aging and wear and tear on the joints, inflammation plays a significant role in its progression. Vitamin C's antioxidant properties may help reduce inflammation and slow the degeneration of cartilage, which is a hallmark of osteoarthritis. Moreover, vitamin C is essential for the synthesis of collagen and other connective tissues, which are crucial for joint health. Some studies have suggested that a diet rich in vitamin C may be associated with a reduced risk of osteoarthritis or a slower disease progression. However, more research is needed to establish a clear link between vitamin C and osteoarthritis prevention or management.

AGE-RELATED MACULAR DEGENERATION

Age-related macular degeneration (AMD) is a leading cause of vision loss in older adults. It is characterized by the deterioration of the macula, a part of the retina responsible for central vision. Oxidative stress and inflammation are believed to contribute to the development and progression of AMD. Vitamin C, with its antioxidant properties, can potentially protect the retina from oxidative damage and reduce the risk of AMD. Some studies have suggested that a diet rich in vitamin C and other antioxidants may be associated with a lower risk of AMD. However, while there is some evidence supporting the role of vitamin C in AMD prevention, further research is necessary to determine its effectiveness in slowing disease progression or managing AMD.

Vitamin C is a versatile nutrient with antioxidant properties that may play a role in preventing and managing chronic diseases such as cardiovascular diseases, cancer, osteoarthritis, and age-related macular degeneration. However, the relationship between vitamin C and these diseases is complex and multifaceted, and more research is needed to establish definitive recommendations for its use in disease prevention and management. In the meantime, maintaining a balanced diet rich in fruits and vegetables, which are natural sources of vitamin C, remains a prudent approach to support overall health and potentially reduce the risk of chronic diseases.

CHAPTER TEN

VITAMIN C AND MENTAL HEALTH

ROLE IN BRAIN HEALTH

Vitamin C, also known as ascorbic acid, is widely recognized for its role in supporting overall health, but its significance extends to mental well-being and brain health as well. This essential nutrient plays a crucial role in several key processes within the brain. One of its primary functions is its powerful antioxidant properties, which help protect brain cells from oxidative stress and damage caused by free radicals. Oxidative stress has been linked to various neurodegenerative disorders, and vitamin C's antioxidant capabilities may help reduce the risk of such conditions.

Furthermore, vitamin C is necessary for the synthesis of neurotransmitters like dopamine and serotonin, which are essential for regulating mood and emotional stability. Adequate levels of these neurotransmitters are crucial for maintaining mental health. A deficiency in vitamin C can disrupt the delicate balance of these chemicals, potentially leading to mood swings, irritability, and even symptoms of depression and anxiety.

Depression and anxiety are common mental health disorders that affect millions of individuals worldwide. Emerging research has shed light on the potential role of vitamin C in managing and preventing these conditions. As mentioned earlier, vitamin C is involved in the synthesis of neurotransmitters, and an imbalance in these chemicals can contribute to the development of mood disorders like depression and anxiety.

Low levels of vitamin C have been associated with an increased risk of depression. This association may be due to the impact of vitamin C on the regulation of cortisol, a stress hormone. Elevated cortisol levels are often observed in individuals with depression and anxiety, and vitamin C can help modulate these levels, potentially reducing the severity of these conditions.

Moreover, vitamin C's antioxidant properties play a role in protecting the brain against oxidative stress, which is often elevated in individuals with depression and anxiety. Reducing oxidative stress can help mitigate the damage to brain cells and may improve symptoms in those suffering from mood disorders.

It's important to note that while vitamin C can be a valuable component of a holistic approach to managing depression and anxiety, it is not a standalone treatment. It should be integrated into a comprehensive treatment plan that may include therapy, medication, lifestyle modifications, and other therapeutic interventions.

COGNITIVE DECLINE

Cognitive decline, characterized by deterioration in memory, thinking, and reasoning skills, is a significant concern as people age. Alzheimer's disease and other forms of dementia are the most extreme manifestations of cognitive decline. While the causes of cognitive decline are multifaceted, the potential role of vitamin C in maintaining cognitive function is worth exploring.

Vitamin C's antioxidant properties are particularly important in the context of cognitive health. Oxidative stress and inflammation are associated with the development and progression of neurodegenerative diseases.

Vitamin C's ability to neutralize free radicals and reduce oxidative stress can contribute to the protection of brain cells, potentially slowing down cognitive decline.

Additionally, vitamin C plays a role in the synthesis of neurotransmitters, which are essential for optimal brain function. The production and regulation of neurotransmitters are vital for memory, learning, and overall cognitive performance. Deficiencies in vitamin C may disrupt these processes, potentially contributing to cognitive impairment.

While research on vitamin C's direct impact on cognitive decline is ongoing, it is generally recommended to maintain a balanced diet rich in antioxidants like vitamin C, as part of a broader strategy for preserving cognitive function in aging individuals.

However, it's essential to consider other factors, such as physical activity, mental stimulation, and social engagement, in promoting cognitive health and preventing cognitive decline.

Vitamin C plays a multifaceted role in mental health and brain function. It's antioxidant properties, influence on neurotransmitter synthesis, and potential impact on mood disorders and cognitive decline underscore the importance of ensuring an adequate intake of this essential nutrient.

CHAPTER ELEVEN

VITAMIN C AND ATHLETES

EXERCISE AND OXIDATIVE STRESS

Exercise is a crucial component of an athlete's routine, but it also comes with a potential downside: oxidative stress. During intense physical activity, the body's oxygen consumption increases dramatically. This elevated oxygen consumption can lead to the production of reactive oxygen species (ROS), which are highly reactive molecules that can damage cells and tissues. This phenomenon, often referred to as oxidative stress, can result in muscle fatigue, and inflammation, and even impair an athlete's performance.

Vitamin C, also known as ascorbic acid, plays a pivotal role in mitigating oxidative stress. It is a powerful antioxidant that can neutralize ROS, thereby reducing their damaging effects on the body. Athletes, particularly those engaged in strenuous and endurance activities, may experience increased oxidative stress. Therefore, maintaining adequate levels of vitamin C in their diet can be beneficial for counteracting this stress and supporting overall well-being.

The benefits of vitamin C for athletes extend beyond its role in combating oxidative stress. This essential micronutrient offers several advantages that can directly impact an athlete's performance and recovery.

1. Immune Support: Intense training can temporarily weaken the immune system, making athletes susceptible to infections. The benefits of vitamin C on the immune system are widely recognized. It helps in the production of white blood cells, which are vital for fighting off infections and

illnesses, and it can also reduce the duration and severity of colds.

2. Collagen Synthesis: Collagen is a structural protein that forms the connective tissues in the body, including tendons and ligaments. Vitamin C is essential for collagen synthesis, which is crucial for maintaining healthy joints and reducing the risk of injuries for athletes.

3. Wound Healing: Injuries and muscle tears are common in sports. Vitamin C plays a critical role in the body's natural wound-healing process. It aids in the repair and

regeneration of damaged tissues, facilitating a quicker recovery.

4. Iron Absorption: Iron is essential for oxygen transport in the blood. Non-heme iron, which is the kind of iron included in plant-based diets, is better absorbed when vitamin C is present. This is particularly relevant for athletes following vegetarian or vegan diets, as they may be at a higher risk of iron deficiency.

DOSAGE AND TIMING

The recommended daily allowance (RDA) for vitamin C varies depending on factors like age, sex, and pregnancy status. For adult men, it's about 90 milligrams, and for adult women, it's 75 milligrams. However, athletes, especially those engaged in rigorous training, may require higher doses to reap the benefits of vitamin C fully.

The timing of vitamin C consumption is also crucial. It's generally advisable to maintain a consistent intake throughout the day. Athletes can include vitamin C-rich foods in their meals and snacks. Common sources of vitamin C include citrus fruits (oranges, grapefruits), strawberries, kiwi, and vegetables like broccoli, bell peppers, and kale.

Supplementation is another option, and some athletes choose to take vitamin C supplements. The appropriate dosage should be determined based on individual needs, and it's wise to consult with a healthcare professional to determine the right dose for your specific requirements.

Vitamin C is a valuable micronutrient for athletes due to its role in combating oxidative stress, supporting the immune system, aiding collagen synthesis, promoting wound healing, and enhancing iron absorption.

The dosage and timing of vitamin C intake should be tailored to the individual's nutritional needs and training intensity. A well-balanced diet rich in vitamin C sources is an excellent way for athletes to ensure they receive the numerous benefits this essential vitamin has to offer.

CHAPTER TWELVE

RISKS AND SIDE EFFECTS

SIDE EFFECTS OF HIGH DOSES

High doses of various substances, whether they are medications, supplements, or even certain foods, can lead to a range of adverse side effects. These adverse effects are generally more apparent and potentially harmful when compared to conventional or recommended doses. The risk of suffering side effects increases as the dose surpasses the recommended level. One typical type of chemical where large doses might lead to negative effects is prescription medications.

When patients exceed the specified amount of a medicine, they may experience adverse effects such as nausea, vomiting, dizziness, and headaches. These side effects might vary in strength, and their severity typically relies on the individual medication in question. High doses of opioids, for example, can lead to respiratory depression, a potentially life-threatening illness. Furthermore, the continued use of large doses of pharmaceuticals can result in drug tolerance, addiction, and withdrawal symptoms, which can exacerbate the issue further.

High amounts of vitamins and minerals, commonly taken in the form of supplements, can also cause negative effects. For instance, excess vitamin C can lead to digestive troubles, while high amounts of vitamin D can result in hypocalcaemia, a condition defined by higher levels of calcium in the blood, potentially causing kidney stones and other health concerns. It's vital to contact a healthcare provider before using any dietary supplements to avoid exceeding acceptable dosage limits.

Additionally, large quantities of certain recreational substances, such as alcohol or illicit narcotics, can have severe and immediate negative effects. For instance, excessive alcohol consumption can lead to alcohol poisoning, which can be life-threatening. Similarly, excessive doses of illicit narcotics can cause hallucinations, convulsions, heart arrhythmias, and even death.

Large quantities of numerous substances, including prescriptions, supplements, and recreational drugs, can lead to a wide range of side effects, which may vary in severity and might represent major health hazards. It is vital to follow suggested dosages and speak with a healthcare practitioner to avoid these possibly hazardous outcomes.

ALLERGIES AND SENSITIVITIES

Allergies and sensitivities are individual reactions to certain chemicals that the immune system labels as harmful, even though they could be innocuous to others. Allergic responses and sensitivities can appear in a variety of ways, ranging from minor discomfort to life-threatening scenarios. Understanding these reactions is critical in determining the risks and side effects associated with exposure to allergens.

Allergic reactions generally involve the release of histamines and other immune system chemicals, resulting in symptoms such as itching, hives, sneezing, runny nose, watery eyes, or gastrointestinal difficulties. These reactions can occur in response to a wide range of allergens, including specific foods, insect stings, pollen, pet dander, and numerous medications.

In severe situations, allergic responses can develop into anaphylaxis, a life-threatening illness that causes a rapid drop in blood pressure, swelling of the throat, and trouble breathing. This requires rapid medical attention, as it can be lethal without prompt intervention.

Sensitivities, on the other hand, do not include the immune system's quick and acute response but can nevertheless result in uncomfortable or unfavorable reactions. For example, some persons are sensitive to certain meals or food components, including lactose or gluten, resulting in gastrointestinal discomfort. Others may have sensitivities to scents, chemicals, or environmental variables, leading to symptoms such as headaches, skin rashes, or respiratory difficulties.

It's crucial to note that allergies and sensitivities can be extremely individual, and the degree of reactions varies from person to person. Avoiding triggers and, in the case of allergies, keeping epinephrine auto-injectors on hand in case of an anaphylactic reaction are key components of recognizing and managing these reactions.

A wide range of hazards and side effects, from little discomfort to life-threatening circumstances, can be associated with allergies and sensitivities. To reduce these possible hazards and side effects, it is essential to be aware of one's allergies and sensitivities and to take the necessary precautions.

POSSIBLE DANGERS

The uncertainties and risks connected to particular items, situations, or actions are referred to as potential risks. These dangers can take many different forms, such as worries about one's finances, health, safety, or the environment. An essential component of decision-making, both for individuals and organizations, is recognizing and controlling possible risks.

Health risks are a noteworthy subset of potential hazards. Potential dangers in healthcare could be the transmission of infectious diseases, adverse reactions to medical treatments, or difficulties following surgery. Healthcare professionals must evaluate these prospective dangers and take the necessary actions to reduce them while maintaining the highest standards of patient care.

Uncertainties surrounding loans, investments, and economic conditions are all considered financial risks. Businesses and individuals alike need to think about the possible risks involved in their financial decisions. Investing in stocks, for instance, may result in a loss of capital if the market collapses, and taking on a large debt load may expose oneself to financial insolvency in the event of an economic crisis.

About sustainability and climate change, environmental risks are becoming more and more important. Natural disasters, resource depletion, and pollution are some of the dangers involved. Governments and businesses must take into account any possible environmental risks associated with their operations and put policies in place to lessen their ecological footprint and stop environmental harm.

The possible threats in a variety of environments, such as public areas and workplaces, are referred to as safety risks. For example, employers ought to carry out risk assessments to pinpoint possible dangers that can cause mishaps or injuries, and then put safety precautions in place to safeguard staff members and the general public.

CHAPTER THIRTEEN

VITAMIN C AND OTHER NUTRIENTS

Ascorbic acid, another name for vitamin C, is a necessary substance that is essential to several bodily physiological functions. Its capacity to interact with and improve the absorption of certain other nutrients is one of the main factors contributing to its significance. It's critical to talk about how vitamin C interacts with other nutrients in this setting to optimize their effects.

VITAMIN C AND IRON ABSORPTION

It is commonly recognized that vitamin C helps the body absorb iron from food. For our bodies to produce hemoglobin, the protein that carries oxygen in our blood, iron is a necessary mineral. But in contrast to iron obtained from animal sources (heme iron), iron from plant meals (non-heme iron) is less easily absorbed by the body. This is where the role of vitamin C is relevant.

The absorption of non-heme iron from plant sources is enhanced by vitamin C. By doing this, non-heme iron is reduced to a form that is easier to absorb.

This transformation takes place in the stomach, where iron and vitamin C combine to create a complex that the body can easily absorb. Therefore, eating foods high in vitamin C, such as citrus fruits, strawberries, and broccoli, together with plant-based foods high in iron, like spinach, lentils, and beans, can greatly increase the absorption of iron. Due to their increased reliance on non-heme iron sources, people who follow vegetarian or vegan diets should pay special attention to the synergy between vitamin C and iron.

VITAMIN C AND VITAMIN D

The relationship between these two nutrients is more about their combined effects on the immune system and general health than it is about absorption. The immune-stimulating qualities of both vitamins are well established, and they frequently enhance immune function in concert.

The fundamental function of vitamin D is to control the intestinal absorption of calcium, which is essential for bone health. Contrarily, vitamin C strengthens the immune system by encouraging the development of white blood cells, which aid in the body's defense against infections. When it comes to sustaining general well-being, these two vitamins can work in concert with one another. According to certain research, vitamin C can improve the benefits of vitamin D, particularly when it comes to boosting immunological responses. Sustaining an appropriate intake of both vitamins is advantageous for general health, even though the precise processes of their interaction are still not completely understood.

SYNERGISTIC NUTRIENT COMBINATIONS

This idea goes beyond how vitamin C interacts with vitamin D and iron. Numerous nutrients can cooperate to increase their bioavailability in the body. For example, selenium and vitamin E are recognized as synergistic antioxidants, which mean that they work in concert to shield cells from oxidative damage. Flaxseeds and fatty fish, which are high in omega-3 fatty acids, help complement vitamin D in maintaining bone health. Furthermore, appropriate blood coagulation and bone mineralization are ensured by the combined action of calcium and vitamin K.

These complementary nutrient pairings highlight how crucial it is to have a varied and balanced diet. Numerous elements that support general health can be obtained via a diet high in whole grains, lean meats, fruits, and vegetables. People may make educated dietary decisions and guarantee they are getting the most out of their nutrition by being aware of these relationships. It's important to keep in mind that, even though some combinations can improve nutrient absorption and utilization, it's preferable to get the majority of your nutrients from whole foods rather than supplements because the intricate interactions between different nutrients in whole foods are challenging to duplicate in isolated supplements.

CHAPTER FOURTEEN

HOW TO PICK A REPUTABLE SOURCE OF VITAMIN C

There are several important elements to take into account when selecting a high-quality vitamin C supplement to make sure you are obtaining a product that is high-quality, safe, and effective. Reading the product labels is one of the first steps in this procedure. You may learn vital information about the supplement's composition, form, and dose from the material on the label.

Take a look at the ingredients list first. Ascorbic acid or a related type of vitamin C should be included as the primary ingredient in a high-quality vitamin C supplement. Supplements that list a lot of artificial colors, fillers, or ingredients should be avoided. The better the component list is, the more simple and clear it is. In addition, it is helpful to verify the dosage and serving size because these will show you how much vitamin C you are taking in. Make sure the dosage suits your individual dietary and medical requirements.

Third-party testing is another crucial factor to take into account. An impartial laboratory should analyze a reliable supplement to confirm its potency and purity. The product's purported vitamin C content and contamination-free status are verified by independent testing. Seek certifications from groups that demonstrate a dedication to quality and safety, such as Consumer Lab, NSF International, or the United States Pharmacopeia (USP). These organizations carefully evaluate the components and production methods of supplements.

The shelf life and storage of a vitamin C supplement are important considerations as well. Light, heat, and moisture are some of the environmental variables that might cause vitamin C to deteriorate over time. To keep a product safe from light and moisture, look for one that is packaged in an opaque, airtight container and follow the label's storage directions. Furthermore, keep your supplement out of direct sunlight and store it somewhere dry and cool. To make sure the supplement keeps its strength until you complete the bottle, choose one with an acceptable shelf life and pay attention to the product's expiration date.

Choosing a high quality vitamin C supplement requires careful evaluation of the label, independent testing, shelf life, and storage. By understanding the components and dose, you can make sure the supplement meets your needs by reading the labels. Certifications from third-party testing provide further assurance about the potency and purity of the product. Lastly, understanding shelf life and storage conditions will enable you to continue using the vitamin C supplement's usefulness throughout time. By following these steps, you will be able to make an informed decision that benefits your general health and well-being.

CONCLUSION

YUMMY RECIPES TO INCREASE YOUR CONSUMPTION OF VITAMIN C

The role that vitamin C plays in sustaining general health and well-being makes it imperative that you include delectable recipes to increase your intake of this crucial nutrient. Ascorbic acid, another name for vitamin C, is a water-soluble nutrient that is well-known for its many health advantages. Vitamin C is a multifaceted nutrient that serves a multitude of purposes in the body, including immune system support, skin health promotion, and wound healing. It ought to be an essential component of every diet.

Including mouthwatering foods high in vitamin C is not only healthful but also palatable. Several different fruits and vegetables are great providers of this important nutrient. Strawberries, kiwis, guavas, and citrus fruits including oranges, grapefruits, and lemons are all common options. In addition, veggies like broccoli, Brussels sprouts, and bell peppers are excellent choices for your regular meals. Foods high in vitamin C are versatile and make for a delicious and varied culinary experience.

VITAMIN C'S FUNCTION IN YOUR HEALTH

There are many different ways that vitamin C contributes to your health, and one of the most essential ways is by keeping your body robust and resilient. Above all, vitamin C is a strong antioxidant that aids in shielding cells from harm brought on by free radicals. This antioxidant characteristic lowers the danger of chronic illnesses, such as heart problems and some forms of cancer, in addition to aiding in the fight against the indications of age. As a result, include foods high in vitamin C in your diet is a proactive measure to protect your long-term health.

Increasing immunity is one of vitamin C's most well-known effects. It is necessary for the development and operation of white blood cells, which are important immune system constituents. A diet high in vitamin C can help your body fight off infections and heal from illnesses more rapidly, which makes it especially important to take into account the current concerns about world health.

Moreover, collagen synthesis, a protein necessary for the integrity of blood vessels, tendons, ligaments, and skin, depends heavily on vitamin

C. The body is held together by collagen, and your body can properly maintain and repair these structural components if you consume enough vitamins C. This maintains the overall integrity of your body's connective tissues and encourages youthful, supple skin.

It is also well-recognized that vitamin C can lower the chance of developing chronic illnesses like heart disease by preserving normal cholesterol and blood pressure levels. It might also help lower internal inflammation, which is a major contributing cause to several chronic illnesses.

www.ingramcontent.com/pod-product-compliance
Lightning Source LLC
Chambersburg PA
CBHW050920260726

48660CB00001B/317